THE 21 DAY JUICE FAST | HEALTHILY DRINK YOUR WAY THIN

CONGRATULATIONS ON YOUR DECISION TO GET HEALTHY!

The "21" Day Juice Fast
(Healthily Drink Your Way Thin)

COOKBOOK IV

A guide to a *new eating plan* that is not a "DIET", created based on personal experience to help you *finally* achieve your weight loss and health goals.

ALSO BY KYLA LATRICE, MBA

"New Me, New You! (How I Overcame Obesity)"

"The 7 Day Smoothie Detox"

"The 21 Day Slushie & Juice Fast"

"The 21 Day Salad Fast"

"Eat Well and Stay Thin (Living a Healthy You)"

"21 Days to a New Healthy You! Hearty Vegan & Vegetarian Slow Cooker Recipes"

"Twenty-One Healthy Ice Pop Snack Recipes"

"21 Days of Everyday Healthy Snack Recipes"

"All Natural Soups & Stews"

"A Collection of My Favorite Health Recipes"

"A New You! Workout Workbook"

THE "21" DAY JUICE FAST
Healthily Drink Your Way Thin

A 21 DAY JUICE FAST TO RESET YOUR HEALTH, MIND, BODY, METABOLISM AND *"LIFE"*

KYLA LATRICE, MBA

Lady Mirage Publications, Inc.

New York   Memphis   Los Angeles   London   Cape Town   Toronto
Atlanta   Singapore   Japan

Copyright © 2014 by Ms. Kyla Latrice, Inc.
The author is represented by Lady Mirage Literary Agency, Inc.
All rights reserved. In accordance with the U.S. Copyright Act of 1976, the scanning, uploading, and electronic sharing of any part of this book without the permission of the publisher is unlawful piracy and theft of the author's intellectual property. If you would like to use material from the book (other than for review purposes), prior written permission must be obtained by contacting the publisher at
www.LadyMirageAgency.com
Thank you for your support of the author's rights.

Published by:
Lady Mirage Publications, Inc.
3724 Goodman Rd W, Unit 575
Horn Lake, MS 38637
www.LadyMirageAgency.com

Manufactured in the United States of America
First Edition: July 2014

Lady Mirage Publications, Inc. is an imprint and subsidiary of Lady Mirage Global. The Lady Mirage Publications, Inc. name and logo are trademarks of Lady Mirage Global.

Authors within the Lady Mirage Global (under Lady Mirage Agency, Inc.), Lady Mirage Publications and Lady Mirage Literary Agency speakers division provides a wide range of authors for speaking engagements. To find out more information, go to
www.LadyMirageAgency.com
Cover photo provided by www.FreeDigitalPhotos.net
The publisher is not responsible for websites (or their content) that are not owned by the publisher.

Library of Congress Cataloging-in-Publication Data:
eISBN: 978-1-31-075056-4; Print ISBN: 978-0-9975371-3-0
Tennin, Kyla Latrice.
The 21 Day Juice Fast   Pages cm; copyrighted materials.
1.   Health-Nutrition-Diet-Fitness. 2. Cooking. 3. Fitness.
Library of Congress Catalog Card Number: 2016907238

Print Book Edition, License Note

This book is licensed for your personal enjoyment only. This book may not be re-sold or given away to other people. If you would like to share this book with another person, please purchase an additional copy for each recipient.
If you're reading this book and did not purchase it, or it was not purchased for your use only, then please return to your favorite book retailer and purchase your own copy. Thank you for respecting the hard work of this author.

Also Note

In this book, Ms. Latrice begins by explaining a *fast* that she has created, tested and tried, which contributed to her weight loss, weight management and healthy eating lifestyle journey. She has also written this book due to there being so many books, health, weight-loss and "diet" programs currently on the global market. The programs and books she has seen and reviewed are too long, too thick, have too much information and many times, are difficult for people to read. This book was written to ***simplify and shorten*** how to lose weight and maintain your health, for life. It is based on personal experience and is still done today. It's an effective solution.

The "21" Day Juice Fast
(Healthily Drink Your Way Thin)

TABLE OF CONTENTS

SLUSHIES & JUICES RECIPES...40

Day 1: The Carrot Juicer………………...…..……………….42
      Day 2: Watermelon Apple Slush..…..……………..44
Day 3: The Beta-Carotene Juicer……………………46
      Day 4: Pomegranate-Blueberry Slush…..………..…48
Day 5: The Pineapple-Carotene Juicer……....…………50
      Day 6: Watermelon Pineapple Slush..……………52
Day 7: The Spinach-Carotene Juicer…..….………….54
      Day 8: "Myrtle-Beach" Cucumber Slush…..……….56
Day 9: The Cucumber-Beat Apple Juicer..…………….58
      Day 10: White Grape Slush………….……………60
Day 11: The Apple-Cucumber Juicer………………….62
      Day 12: Peach Grape Watermelon Slush...………..64
Day 13: The Celery-Cucumber Juicer………………….66
      Day 14: Pineapple Red-Grape Slush…....…..……..68
Day 15: The Orange-Beat Juicer……………………..70
      Day 16: Watermelon Acai-Berry Slush…..….……...72
Day 17: The Cucumber-Beat Juicer…………...……..74
      Day 18: "Go-Green" Apple Slush……………..……76
Day 19: The Pear-Beat Juicer………....……..……..78
      Day 20: Lemon-Lime Pear Slush…………….……80
Day 21: The Lemon-Beat Juicer………….……………82

INDEX…………………………………………....84
      Slushies & Juices Recipes………..…..……..84

DEDICATION

This cookbook is dedicated to men and women around the world that have dealt with or are beginning to deal with food addiction, obesity and/or declining health.

I also dedicate this book to those whom have been "Mirage's" in life; overlooked, betrayed, not good enough, slandered, mistreated, misunderstood, misrepresented and even treated unfairly because of their weight or how they looked on the *outside* to others, when in fact, on the *inside* there's greater.

This new cookbook is also dedicated to men and women around the world that want to
shift from being ordinary to extraordinary and accomplishing what others said you would never be able to do again or never be able to do at all.

Here's to the New You!

ACKNOWLEDGMENTS

I want to **say thank you** to anyone whom has ever betrayed, rejected, mistreated, teased, and misused or looked down upon me. You helped me become GREATER and launched me into my destiny.

Whenever someone throws bricks at you, use them to *"build"*. Build something greater; even your mansion.

And whenever you face opposition, "know" that it is actually an opportunity; a set-back for a set-up to secure the victory, rejection for rewards, pain for gain, lack for prosperity to leave a legacy, misery for miracles and put downs for promotion.

IT'S YOUR TIME…*to bounce back!*

Let's Get Healthy!

AUTHOR'S NOTE

The 21 Day Slushie & Juice Fast (The 21 Juice Fast)
Copyright © 2014
Ms. Kyla Latrice, Inc.
All Rights Reserved.

AFFIDAVIT

All content written herein is of opinion, from personal experience and of suggestion. Individual juice fast and new eating plan results may vary from person to person and no results are guaranteed.

You must put forth effort and do the work necessary to take charge of changing your life and **losing weight**. I did and so can you.

You can also utilize this cookbook if you have already met your weight loss goals and just want to stay healthy with recipes that will keep your metabolism in check and body running smoothly.

Be sure to wash all fruits, vegetables, foods, etc. thoroughly before beginning any new
eating or meal plan.

ALL RIGHTS RESERVED

No portion of this publication may be reproduced, stored in any electronic system, or transmitted in any form by any means; electronic, mechanical,
photocopy, recording or otherwise, without written permission from the author.

Brief quotations may be used in literary reviews with the consent of the author and publisher.

"ON-THE-GO"

This cookbook *(and all of my cookbooks, books, workbook and manuals)* can be read and applied in airports, on trains, at work on your lunch break, in grocery stores while shopping for and planning your weekly meals, at bookstore cafes, at restaurants *(for quick decision making; to remember your health and/or weight loss goals)* and even in shopping malls.

In addition, *this book can be brought to* fast food restaurants (to pull up and look through to remember your goals before ordering), at the park (before a jog or potluck), during your hotel stays, on vacations and at airport food counters when ordering your meals and drinks *(so you remember your goals and what to eat and drink)*.

This cookbook has been made available on mobile devices via Adobe Digital Editions and DRM (Digital Rights Management).

WORLD STATISTICS

Obesity and Childhood Obesity
Centers for Disease Control and Prevention
http://www.cdc.gov/obesity/data/adult.html
http://www.cdc.gov/nchs/fastats/obesity-overweight.htm

Harvard School of Public Health
http://www.hsph.harvard.edu/obesity-prevention-source/obesity-trends/

World Health Organization
http://www.who.int/topics/obesity/en/

Stroke Awareness and Prevention
http://www.cdc.gov/stroke/facts.htm

Diabetes Awareness and Prevention
Centers for Disease Control and Prevention
http://www.cdc.gov/diabetes/data/statistics/2014statisticsreport.html

American Diabetes Association
http://www.diabetes.org/diabetes-basics/statistics/

"FASTING"

WHAT IS FASTING?

- Fasting is abstaining from PLEASURABLE foods for a certain amount of time to FOCUS on things that are more important than pleasurable foods to get to the root of what is causing your poor health, obesity, relationships and quality of life.

- It is not a hunger strike.

- You're able to see into your life better and rid it of the bad when you pull away from portion after portion at the dinner table, lunch buffet after buffet with friends and co-workers, nightly binge eating and drinking (whether alcohol, sodas, sugary drinks and the like) and dessert or movie nights on the sofa with a large pizza box and donuts.

- Fasting helps you pinpoint where you overdo things (overindulge), gets you back on track and teaches you how to eat, "in moderation" (balance), for your health and for a better life.

- Your body may not like eating healthy for the first few days (especially if you have never fasted before), but it will adjust.

REASONS FOR FASTING:

- It produces a physical discipline (especially for how, when, where and *what* you eat).

- It rids the body of toxins (just like exercise does when you sweat); cleansing your body and digestive tracts, improving your health and weight.

> Note: If you are on medication, consult your physician before any *fast*.

THE 21 DAY JUICE FAST | HEALTHILY DRINK YOUR WAY THIN

BENEFITS OF FASTING:

- It strengthens *you* and your body.

- Fasting brings joy, happiness and *energy* to your life; and fruits, vegetables, oils, etc. are quite inexpensive. Make a list and shop for your ingredients before you begin.

- You become very aware of *what* and *how much* you eat. You also begin to pay more attention to when and where you always eat/drink and what leads you to OVEREATING.

- Fasting brings humility, revelation and an overall healthy lifestyle (mind, emotions, intellect, etc.).

TYPICAL TYPES OF FASTS:
Sometimes people fast the following from their lives:
- Television (even the internet, social media or video games) for one day, three days or even one week, television during certain hours of the day (to break a cycle of watching certain shows they may be addicted to (like food) that aren't good for them.
  ….or
- To break a cycle of "certain foods" they may eat while watching certain television shows.

- Fasting to abstain from all pleasurable foods and red meats, eating only fruits, vegetables, clear soups, cereals (no white sugar), water, diluted fruit juices (100% juices only) and/or grains.

- Some people even fast people (bad acquaintances, friendships or relationships), leading eventually to moving away from those person's completely, for a better life and health. Your health is your life.

- Many people fast for 24 hours, three days, seven days, 14 days, 21 days or longer. My success and learning my body as well as other persons bodies (whom have fasted when I have fasted) has come from "closely monitoring" how the body reacts to each of these fasts (particularly "21 days") and I've noticed some things and have sculpted recipes to help others find that tremendous success in many areas of their lives as well.

- Fasts should always be broken slowly, especially if you have been on an "extended fast" (a fast for more than 30 days, a salad only fast, a smoothie only fast or even a clear soup only fast).

- Gradually get back into "regular food", until you can completely commit to "healthy food" (and a regular healthy lifestyle); such as having juices for a couple of days, then fruits, vegetables, grains and adding meats back into your diet last, if applicable.

- Typically, people have six meals per day (three main meals (breakfast, lunch and dinner) and three snacks). For each of my Fasts or Recipes, you determine how many meals. Don't worry, fruits and vegetables do not cause obesity, they prevent it. Yet, always watch your portion sizes, in general, and with soups, stews and anything that has meat included. Never eat meat in excess.

- You can even choose to eat one meal per day for 21 days (there are enough recipes listed in this book), a snack, have 5-8 bottles of water and be sure to get a nap in and some exercise during the week. As you advance you can mix your salad fast with a smoothie fast and detox fast by doing one of the fasts, each per week, for 21 days, etc.

THE *"JUICE FAST"* BIRTH

Kyla Latrice is a native of Marks, MS and enjoys food and traveling. Being from a small town and a country gal, she set her goals high. Graduating from a private institution with a Bachelor of Arts Degree (BA) *(women's studies and health background; pre-medicine)* and a Master's Degree (MBA) in Business Administration with **Executive Education at Harvard and Stanford** along with several certifications and nearly 50-80 self-study coursework in legal, intellectual property and self-help, she has become one of the leading entrepreneurs of her time.

Currently Ms. Latrice is finishing up her Doctoral Honorary Degree ***(Doctor of Management in Organizational Leadership)*** and continues to serve on Board of Directors throughout the world for various causes; still relating to her life's purpose and corporations work. Ms. Latrice travels extensively for speaking engagements in the areas of health, wellness, obesity, poverty, domestic violence, branding, image, leadership, mentoring, business, entrepreneurship and the like.

To date, Ms. Latrice has mentored with over 20 plus organizations *(from elementary to senior citizen)*, helping others overcome issues she has faced.

With her first *corporate* job opportunity being at a "Health Food Restaurant" *(when she was age 15 or 16)* to work as a deli attendant at the deli bar, hostess *(when others were out for the day)* and bakery attendant as well as a chef in the *salad bar*.

Her main role was to attend to the deli, to prepare healthy pasta salads, healthy sandwiches, healthy shakes, healthy sundaes and *healthy smoothies*. However, Ms. Latrice was blessed with the opportunity to be called upon whenever management needed her help in the other areas as well, **to continue learning**. This gave Ms. Latrice very valuable experience and a "look" into health and business ownership, a bit deeper, which still remains with her today.

THE *"JUICE FAST"* BIRTH

KYLA LATRICE
BEFORE
21 DAY JUICE FASTS

Ms. Latrice's *(on the left in the photo)* Corporations are inclusive of health restaurants, retail stores, property and land as well as product development organizations along with nonprofit foundations to care for the displaced, homeless.

Further, Ms. Latrice's love for food turned into obesity when her life took a turn in the early 2000's during domestic violence, sinful relationships, bad friendships, emotional binge eating and more; then again in the 2000's with another domestic violence relationship, obesity slander from family members, mental and spiritual abuse, abortion, home foreclosure, vehicle repossession and much *more*, which all have an effect on health, but she made sure her Corporations still stood; to help others.

THE *"JUICE FAST"* BIRTH

KYLA LATRICE
"IN THE MIDDLE"
AFTER GAINING WEIGHT BACK FOR A SECOND TIME
21 DAY JUICE FASTS

THE *"JUICE FAST"* BIRTH

KYLA LATRICE
AFTER
21 DAY JUICE FASTS

THE FINALE

Many factors can contribute to obesity, such as abuse *(mental, spiritual, physical, sexual)*, poor eating habits, environment, bad friendships as well as sin. Personally, I, myself, was never taught how to eat, I did not know what to eat *(that was truly healthy for me)* and I did not know how to deal with life's problems.

Nevertheless, how can someone teach you what they don't know? My first encounter with obesity was when I was a model and went from a size 0 to a size 20/22, **weighing close to 300 pounds** *(then I lost nearly 115 pounds after prayer and seeking a remedy)*.

The second encounter was when I gained some of the first encounters weight back and went from a size 14/16 to a size 4/6 and fitting a 7/8 in jeans, losing 68 pounds. Today, I am going to share my secrets to success with you *(the birth of the "21 Day Salad Fast")* and how I made it out over the years ***and*** kept the weight off. Let's get started and healthy, for life!

GETTING HEALTHY
LIFESTYLE CHANGE

THE 21 DAY JUICE FAST | HEALTHILY DRINK YOUR WAY THIN

Prepare to lose weight on the "Juice Fast" (this is not a "diet", this is an "eating plan" to reprogram your mind, body and metabolism about how to eat (portion control) and regarding what foods you should and should not be eating). It is designed to help you become healthier. Before starting this fast and any of my eating *plans ("The 21 Day Smoothie Fast" and "The 21 Day Salad Fast" as well as "Soups and Stews"),* allow yourself "one week" to prepare for the fast and eating plan by removing the following from your life:

- Negative relationships and friendships; they block you from doing well in life and succeeding, when people begin to see you doing well, they tend to not like it. Choose friendships and associations wisely. Be creative.

- Bad acquaintances; they will eventually want what you have and will cause betrayal to take place in your life through a "set-up" to sabotage all of your hard work. Always keep moving forward.

- Remove the following (slowly) from your daily meals (eating habits) because they contribute to weight gain (some quicker than others): soda, breads, pastas, candy bars and the like and eating second, third and fourth portions of your food. You only need one portion. Don't eat the rest!

- Replace all sodas with diet soda until you can cut soda out of your daily meal plan completely; only drink soda if absolutely necessary *(a lemon-lime beverage)* because there is nothing else to drink. For example, while traveling.

- Remove all "junk food" (cakes, pies, chips, all kinds of desserts and the like) from your kitchen.

- For breads, certain kinds make the weight gain skyrocket; be careful about pizza. Pasta should be limited just like soda, having it only if absolutely necessary, but once every 2-4 months is okay, just like donuts, to stay **balanced** and give your body a break from always eating healthy.

- Again, you only need one portion of food, per meal, work on this and you'll see results quicker.

- Increase your water intake to 5-8 bottled waters a day; bring a bottle with you everywhere you go so you'll be forced to drink it *(instead of something else)* and will program your body to like it *(whether you like it frozen, warm or cold)*.

- When you're out to eating with others, begin selecting items from menus that help *(not hinder)* your **new eating plan**, for example, order a "grilled chicken wrap with a side salad and small water" instead of a double cheeseburger, french fries and large soda. Never super-size, it wastes your results and time spent on improving your health.

- If you have not already, purchase my books: *"The 21 Day Smoothie Fast"* and *"The 21 Day Salad Fast"* to begin, to continue your weight loss and new you.

- And again, remember, commit to single portion eating, eating smaller portions (always have more vegetables on your plate than poultry/ meat), and increase your water intake *(remember to use the restroom)*. Let's begin.

GETTING HEALTHY
SET GOALS

Feel free to purchase my "A New Healthy You Workout Workbook" *(to go with your **new eating plan** and my "fasts" cookbooks* or a composition notebook from any retailer to make your own journal to measure the following (even if you need to do so at your primary care physician's office, a free clinic or go to a free health assessment machine in a retail store location that has one):

Record a written record of each:

- Your Cholesterol Level
- Blood Pressure and Vision Check
- Your actual Height Weight, Height, Bust/Chest and Hips size (write down your goals of where you want to be in the next week, three months, six months and year)
- Record your weight, chest/bust, hips and waist size every Saturday morning at 7am
- Stroll through a department store and notate clothing (or take a camera phone photo) you plan on fitting into someday and notate your current sizes and then return in three months to see how you're fairing up towards your goals
- Pick up my **"A New Healthy You Workout Workbook"** or list in your journal, your reasons for losing weight, changing your life and changing your eating habits

THE 21 DAY JUICE FAST | HEALTHILY DRINK YOUR WAY THIN

- Your BMI (Body Mass Index) and where you are versus where you're supposed to be for your height, weight, age and gender.
- Bottles of "cold water" listed in the recipes section of this book are in reference to drinking 4-5 bottles of 16 fl oz bottles of water, which is equivalent to 8-10 glasses of water per day.
- Water is vital for living and for being healthy.
- The amount of water within the human body is typically 50-65% water and in infants, 78%.
- Water assists your body with digesting food and getting nutrients from the foods you have eaten to your blood, brain and other parts of your body, in order to function; emptying the body of waste and toxins, helps deliver oxygen to the body, helps prevent constipation and even regulates body temperature (in your cells, organs and tissues).

A (BMI) Chart is below for your convenience.

BMI	<(less than) 18.5	=	Underweight
BMI	18.5-24.9	=	Normal Weight
BMI	25-29.9	=	Overweight
BMI	>(more than) 30	=	Obese

GETTING HEALTHY
WHILE TRAVELING

If you'll be traveling by airplane, helicopter or private jet (smile):

- ➢ Research where you will be eating ahead of time (food choices, ingredients and prices).
- ➢ Bring bottled water.
- ➢ Resist vending machines and relying of fast food at your final destination.
- ➢ Bring your own snacks (trail mix, cashews, a banana, apple slices, peanuts) and
- ➢ Workout for free in your hotel room, taking the stairs instead of elevators and walking at the Mall.

If traveling by car:

- ➢ Pack your own cooler with ice for your bottled waters, fruits and raw vegetables.
- ➢ Consider bringing a bag of oranges & any other food that can be eaten warm or cold on the road.

If you'll be traveling by bus, train, or other means:

- ➢ Research where you will be eating ahead of time (food choices, ingredients and prices).
- ➢ Bring bottled water.
- ➢ Bring your own snacks (trail mix, cashews, a banana, apple slices, peanuts for the long trip) and
- ➢ Bring something to read or play, to keep your mind off of food and *fictious* hunger.
- ➢ At your destination, stand more than you sit (to keep your body moving) and since you have been sitting during traveling for your trip.

Juicers and Blenders, Examples & Where to Purchase
AMAZON.COM
http://www.amazon.com/b?node=3241811011 (Centrifugal Juicers are the best on the market; Purchase a Juicer according to your monetary budget and style)

http://www.amazon.com/Kuvings-NJ-9500U-Centrifugal-Extractor-Silver/dp/B005G05JJ6/ref=sr_1_37?s=kitchen&ie=UTF8&qid=1426006281&sr=1-37 (Kuvings Centrifugal Juicers)

http://www.amazon.com/juicers/b?ie=UTF8&node=289926 (All Juicer Types, including Citrus)

http://www.amazon.com/MaxiMatic-EPB-2572-Elite-Cuisine-Personal/dp/B008GS8PRI/ref=sr_1_23?s=kitchen&ie=UTF8&qid=1426007484&sr=1-23 (Sample On-The-Go Mixer)

AMAZON JUICERS
www.amazon.com

Photo Credit: Kuvings Brand

GETTING HEALTHY
YOUR NEW WORKOUT PLAN

During my both times of being obese, I never worked out at a gym nor went outside of my home to run *(weighing in at 278 pounds and trying to start my "new me" as a jogger was terrible on my knees)* to lose weight, I did it all at home, on the floor, in a compact room, near a closet. I suggest you begin a "workout regime" by doing simple workouts, such as crunches, stretching, leg lifts and a few push-ups.

Everyone cannot do cardio in the gym (paid membership prices or because of lack of transportation), running outside or bouncing around in-doors for 1-3 hours like actors and actresses on television, whom are likely being ***paid monetary*** compensation or by other means to film the infomercial.

Remain constant and do this 3-4 times a week, for 15-35 minutes each day. On your workout OFF days, do 100 crunches before going to bed. Consider purchasing my "Workout Workbook" to keep up with your Fitness Plan. In addition, you burn calories when you sleep, by drinking water, by exercising (which helps you live longer as well) and by **movement** (whether your arms, legs, looking out of a window, etc.).

Furthermore, water helps break down food and helps food digest. Your can also do a "mental workout" by cutting out negative people, places and things from your life.

You'll find that you have more peace in your brain and life, when you replace them with reading inspirational books, movies, community work and exercise or things you love, such as knitting, a ball game, taking a site seeing road trip (alone) every now and then or mentoring someone.

Notes

THE SIX MONTH RULE
GIVE IT *"TIME"*

THE SIX-MONTH RULE

On a 21-Day Salad Fast, weight [pounds] have been known to drop quickly for many people. However, the goal here is to also keep the weight off. Stay focused and be committed to at least six-months of "health work".

Remember to journal your progress.

There's something about when you write things down, they get *ACCOMPLISHED!* Also give yourself a total of six-months to work on your "New You" simply because you may lose inches first and not weight, until your weight catches up with your inches (this is what took place with me; loosing 10-12 pounds per month).

Inches first then one day the weight just fell off. And for others, sometimes weight first, then inches.

GO BACK TO THE DEPARTMENT STORE

Revisit those same department stores that you went to on the first week of your new lifestyle change, try on new clothing sizes to see where you are with your goals.

I suggest that you "mentally shop" for a new suit, a dinner dress, clothing for you next vacation (Hawaii maybe), your first pair of skinny jeans or baseball gear to wear to a game; all after you have reached your goals; to *CELEBRATE!*

"SLUSHIE & JUICE FAST"
RECIPES

WEEK 1
CARROTS WEEK

Photo Credit: Anusorn Pnachol
FREEDIGITALPHOTOS.NET

WEEK 1, DAY 1
(THE CARROT JUICER)

Day 1 of Week 1: Carrots and Apples

Add 2 whole carrots into a juicer, Add 1 whole apple, Juice until complete, Pour into a glass over ice, if desired or bullet to go blender cup or blender mug, Add ½ cup of chilled 100% orange juice (no pulp), Serve immediately

Health Notes:

Apples – Apples help whiten your teeth by producing saliva, assisting with reducing tooth decay, protects against cancers, gallstones, hemorrhoids, constipation and high cholesterol. They also help you control your weight, prevent cataracts, decrease your chances of developing diabetes and boost your immune system (red apples; which have an antioxidant called quercetin in them). Apples also have Vitamins C, A and Flavonoids, Phosphorus, Iron and Calcium as well as Potassium to help promote heart health.

Carrots - Carrots can be white, yellow, red, purple and orange. They are also great for your teeth, killing off harmful germs in the mouth to help prevent tooth decay. Carrots also have a great source of Vitamin A, beta carotene *(an antioxidant to help maintain healthy skin),* Alkaline elements (which help purify and revitalize the blood) and Potassium *(helping the body maintain normal blood pressure levels).*

Weight Management Tips:
- Drink 4-5 bottles of cold water today.
- Get 7-8 hours of sleep; take a 20 minute nap today.
- Have your Juice as breakfast and after your evening workout for best results.
- Do 100 crunches before going to bed (2 sets, 50 each); to burn calories, flatten or to keep your stomach flattened, to build muscle and burn additional calories as you sleep.

SLUSH

Photo Credit: zirconicusso
FREEDIGITALPHOTOS.NET

WEEK 1, DAY 2
(WATERMELON APPLE SLUSH)

Day 2 of Week 1: Watermelon and Yellow Apples

Add 3 whole watermelon stalks into a blender, Add 2 whole (sliced) apples, Add 1 cup of CRUSHED ice, Blend until thick and smooth, Add ½ cup of chilled 100% apple juice, Pour into a glass or bullet to go blender cup or blender mug, Serve immediately

Health Notes:

Apples – Apples help whiten your teeth by producing saliva, assisting with reducing tooth decay, protects against cancers, gallstones, hemorrhoids, constipation and high cholesterol. They also help you control your weight, prevent cataracts, decrease your chances of developing diabetes and boost your immune system (red apples; which have an antioxidant called quercetin in them). Apples also have Vitamins C, A and Flavonoids, Phosphorus, Iron and Calcium as well as Potassium to help promote heart health.

Watermelon - Watermelon is a plant that is originally from Southern Africa. Its fruit is a special berry that has a ripe source of Vitamins C, A, D, B-12, beta carotene, thiamin and B-6. Iron, Calcium, potassium and magnesium are also included. Watermelon is low in calories and aids in wound healing, stress relief and **quenching cravings** to assist with weight loss.

Weight Management Tips:
- Drink 4-5 bottles of cold water today.
- Get 7-8 hours of sleep and take a 20 minute nap during the day.

THE 21 DAY JUICE FAST | HEALTHILY DRINK YOUR WAY THIN

JUICE

Photo Credit: Anusorn Pnachol
FREEDIGITALPHOTOS.NET

WEEK 1, DAY 3
(THE BETA-CAROTENE JUICER)

Day 3 of Week 1: Beats and Carrots

Add 2 whole carrots into a juicer, Add 1/2 of a beat, Juice until complete, Pour into a glass over ice, if desired or bullet to go blender cup or blender mug, Add ½ cup of chilled 100% cranberry juice, Serve immediately

Health Notes:

Carrots - Carrots can be white, yellow, red, purple and orange. They are also great for your teeth, killing off harmful germs in the mouth to help prevent tooth decay. Carrots also have a great source of Vitamin A, beta carotene *(an antioxidant to help maintain healthy skin)*, Alkaline elements (which help purify and revitalize the blood) and Potassium *(helping the body maintain normal blood pressure levels).*

Beats – Beats cleanse the body and are a tonic for the liver and purifies the blood as well as prevents many forms of cancer. Beats also help reduce depression, high blood pressure, give energy and are a great source of Fiber, Vitamins A, B & C, beta-carotene, Iron, folic acid *(especially for women that are pregnant along with the Vitamin B and Iron)* as well as Potassium and Magnesium. Beats also help you detoxify your body and boost your stamina and bone strength and help fight Alzheimer's disease and inflammation.

Weight Management Tips:
- Drink 4-5 bottles of cold water today.
- Get 7-8 hours of sleep; take a 20 minute nap today.
- Have your Juice as breakfast and after your evening workout for best results.
- Do 100 crunches before going to bed (2 sets, 50 each); to burn calories, flatten or to keep your stomach flattened, to build muscle and burn additional calories as you sleep.

SLUSH

Photo Credit: zirconicusso
FREEDIGITALPHOTOS.NET

WEEK 1, DAY 4
(POMEGRANATE-BLUEBERRY SLUSH)

Day 4 of Week 1: Watermelon, Yellow Apples and Pomegranate-Blueberry Juice

Add 3 whole watermelon stalks into a blender, Add 2 whole (sliced) apples, Add 1 cup of CRUSHED ice, Blend until thick and smooth, Add ½ cup of chilled 100% apple juice, Add ½ cup of Pomegranate-Blueberry Juice, Pour into a glass or bullet to go blender cup or blender mug, Serve immediately

Health Notes:

Watermelon - Watermelon is a plant that is originally from Southern Africa. Its fruit is a special berry that has a ripe source of Vitamins C, A, D, B-12, beta carotene, thiamin and B-6. Iron, Calcium, potassium and magnesium are also included. Watermelon is low in calories and aids in wound healing and reduces cravings to assist with weight loss.

Apples – Apples help whiten your teeth by producing saliva, assisting with reducing tooth decay, protects against cancers, gallstones, hemorrhoids, constipation and high cholesterol. They also help you control your weight, prevent cataracts, decrease your chances of developing diabetes and boost your immune system (red apples; which have an antioxidant called quercetin in them).

Pomegranate – Pomegranate Juice is great for your skin, helps reduce stress, breast and prostate cancer development and heart disease and improves blood flow in the body. This juice also helps maintain good cholesterol levels and fights diabetes, being rich in Vitamins A, C and E and folic acid.

Weight Management Tips:
- Drink 4-5 bottles of cold water today.
- Get 7-8 hours of sleep; take a 20 minute nap today.

JUICE

Photo Credit: Anusorn Pnachol
FREEDIGITALPHOTOS.NET

WEEK 1, DAY 5
(THE PINEAPPLE-CAROTENE JUICER)

Day 5 of Week 1: Carrots and Pineapple

Add 3 whole carrots into a juicer, Add 2 pineapple stalks, Juice until complete, Pour into a glass over ice, if desired or bullet to go blender cup or blender mug, Add ½ cup of chilled 100% apple juice, Serve immediately

Health Notes:

Carrots - Carrots can be white, yellow, red, purple and orange. They are also great for your teeth, killing off harmful germs in the mouth to help prevent tooth decay. Carrots also have a great source of Vitamin A, beta carotene *(an antioxidant to help maintain healthy skin),* Alkaline elements (which help purify and revitalize the blood) and Potassium *(helping the body maintain normal blood pressure levels).*

Pineapples – Today, the largest producers of pineapples are in Brazil, Costa Rica, the United States, Hawaii and the Philippines. Pineapples are a natural weight loss food and are rich in Vitamin C, Thiamin, copper and boost the immune system to fight against colds, flu symptoms and other diseases. They also help ease arthritis pain, are low in calories and are very filling; keeping you fuller longer, to prevent overeating.

Weight Management Tips:
- Drink 4-5 bottles of cold water today.
- Get 7-8 hours of sleep; take a 20 minute nap today.
- Have your Juice as breakfast and after your evening workout for best results.
- Do 100 crunches before going to bed (2 sets, 50 each); to burn calories, flatten or to keep your stomach flattened, to build muscle and burn additional calories as you sleep.

SLUSH

Photo Credit: zirconicusso
FREEDITIALPHOTOS.NET

WEEK 1, DAY 6
(WATERMELON PINEAPPLE SLUSH)

Day 6 of Week 1: Watermelon, Pineapple and Apple Juice

Add 3 whole watermelon stalks into a blender, Add 2 whole pineapple, Add 1 cup of CRUSHED ice, Blend until thick and smooth, Add ½ cup of chilled 100% apple juice, Pour into a glass or bullet to go blender cup or blender mug, Serve immediately

Health Notes:

Watermelon - Watermelon is a plant that is originally from Southern Africa. Its fruit is a special berry that has a ripe source of Vitamins C, A, D, B-12, beta carotene, thiamin and B-6. Iron, Calcium, potassium and magnesium are also included. Watermelon is low in calories and aids in wound healing, stress relief and quenching cravings to assist with weight loss.

Pineapples – Today, the largest producers of pineapples are in Brazil, Costa Rica, the United States, Hawaii and the Philippines. Pineapples are a natural weight loss food and are rich in Vitamin C, Thiamin, copper and boosts the immune system to fight against colds, flu symptoms and other diseases. They also help ease arthritis pain, are low in calories and are very filling; keeping you fuller longer, to prevent overeating.

Weight Management Tips:
- Drink 4-5 bottles of cold water today.
- Get 7-8 hours of sleep and take a 20 minute nap during the day.

THE 21 DAY JUICE FAST | HEALTHILY DRINK YOUR WAY THIN

JUICE

Photo Credit: Anusorn Pnachol
FREEDIGITALPHOTOS.NET

WEEK 1, DAY 7
(THE SPINACH-CAROTENE JUICER)

Day 7 of Week 1: Spinach and Carrots

Add 4 cups of spinach into a juicer, Add 2 whole carrots, Juice until complete, Pour into a glass over ice, if desired or bullet to go blender cup or blender mug, Add ½ cup of chilled 100% white grape juice, Serve immediately

Health Notes:

Carrots - Carrots can be white, yellow, red, purple and orange. They are also great for your teeth, killing off harmful germs in the mouth to help prevent tooth decay. Carrots also have a great source of Vitamin A, beta carotene *(an antioxidant to help maintain healthy skin),* Alkaline elements (which help purify and revitalize the blood) and Potassium *(helping the body maintain normal blood pressure levels).*

Spinach – Spinach are filled with Vitamins C, E, beta-carotene and even zinc. They also have a large amount of Vitamin K *(helping with brain function)* helping the nervous system and fighting stroke and cardiovascular disease. They also help maintain strong bones and prevent excess activation of osteoclasts (cells that break bones down). Spinach also help prevent osteoporosis, high blood pressure, vision problems *(protecting the eyes from cataracts and macular degeneration as you age)* and immune deficiencies.

Weight Management Tips:

- Drink 4-5 bottles of cold water today.
- Get 7-8 hours of sleep; take a 20 minute nap today.
- Have your Juice as breakfast and after your evening workout for best results.
- Do 100 crunches before going to bed (2 sets, 50 each); to burn calories, flatten or to keep your stomach flattened, to build muscle and burn additional calories as you sleep.

WEEK 2
CUCUMBERS WEEK

Photo Credit: zirconicusso
FREEDIGITALPHOTOS.NET

WEEK 2, DAY 8
("MYRTLE-BEACH" WATERMELON CUCUMBER SLUSH)

Day 1 of Week 2: Watermelon and Cucumbers

Add 3 whole watermelon stalks into a blender, Add 1 whole peeled cucumber, Add 1 cup of CRUSHED ice, Blend until thick and smooth, Add ½ cup of chilled 100% apple juice, Pour into a glass or bullet to go blender cup or blender mug, Serve immediately

Health Notes:

Watermelon - Watermelon is a plant that is originally from Southern Africa. Its fruit is a special berry that has a ripe source of Vitamins C, A, D, B-12, beta carotene, thiamin and B-6. Iron, Calcium, potassium and magnesium are also included. Watermelon is low in calories and aids in wound healing, stress relief and **quenching cravings** to assist with weight loss.

Cucumbers – Cucumbers are in the family of melons, squash and pumpkins. They are a great source of Vitamins K, C, A and B and are made up 95% water and are great for the eyes, skin and hair due to their anti-inflammatory properties and hair growth stimulation. They also help fight cancers (ovarian, uterine, breast as well as prostate) and aid in weight loss, digestion, blood pressure control, cholesterol reduction and joint pain relief (that is associated with arthritis). Cucumbers also dissolve kidney stones and rid the body of waste products.

Weight Management Tips:
- Drink 4-5 bottles of cold water today.
- Get 7-8 hours of sleep; take a 20 minute nap today.

THE 21 DAY JUICE FAST | HEALTHILY DRINK YOUR WAY THIN

JUICE

Photo Credit: Anusorn Pnachol
FREEDITIALPHOTOS.NET

WEEK 2, DAY 9
(THE CUCUMBER-BEAT APPLE JUICER)

Day 2 of Week 2: Cucumbers and Beats

Add 2 whole cucumbers into a juicer, Add 1 whole beat, Juice until complete, Pour into a glass over ice, if desired or bullet to go blender cup or blender mug, Add ½ cup of chilled 100% apple juice, Serve immediately

Health Notes:

Beats – Beats cleanse the body and are a tonic for the liver and purifies the blood as well as prevents many forms of cancer. Beats also help reduce depression, high blood pressure, give energy and are a great source of Fiber, Vitamins A, B & C, beta-carotene, Iron, folic acid *(especially for women that are pregnant along with Vitamin B and Iron)* as well as Potassium and Magnesium. Beats also help you detoxify your body and help fight Alzheimer's disease.

Cucumbers – Cucumbers are in the family of melons, squash and pumpkins. They are a great source of Vitamins K, C, A and B and are made up 95% water and are great for the eyes, skin and hair due to their anti-inflammatory properties and hair growth stimulation. They also help fight cancers (ovarian, uterine, breast as well as prostate) and aid in weight loss, digestion, blood pressure control, cholesterol reduction and joint pain relief.

Weight Management Tips:
- Drink 4-5 bottles of cold water today.
- Get 7-8 hours of sleep; take a 20 minute nap today.
- Have your Juice as breakfast and after your evening workout for best results.
- Do 100 crunches before going to bed (2 sets, 50 each); to burn calories, flatten or to keep your stomach flattened, to build muscle and burn additional calories as you sleep.

SLUSH

Photo Credit: zirconicusso
FREEDIGITALPHOTOS.NET

WEEK 2, DAY 10
(THE WHITE GRAPE SLUSH)

Day 3 of Week 2: Grapes, Yellow Apples and Apple Juice

Add 3 cups of white grapes (or green) into a blender, Add 2 whole (sliced) apples, Add 1 cup of CRUSHED ice, Blend until thick and smooth, Add ½ cup of chilled 100% apple juice, Pour into a glass or bullet to go blender cup or blender mug, Serve immediately

Health Notes:

Grapes – Grapes originated from Spain and are berries that are similar to blueberries the most. They are power-packed with Vitamins K, C and ripe antioxidants for boosting your health. Grapes also come in various colors; green (white grapes are green grapes), black, pink, yellow, purple and even red. Grapes also heal brain damage, are good for your heart (so that blood can flow through blood vessels more easily) and reduce the cells' ability to store fat, which make them great for weight loss and weight management. They also help fight diabetes, inflammation, skin diseases and aid in muscle health.

Apples – Apples help whiten your teeth by producing saliva, assisting with reducing tooth decay, protects against cancers, gallstones, hemorrhoids, constipation and high cholesterol. They also help you control your weight, prevent cataracts, decrease your chances of developing diabetes and boost your immune system (red apples; which have an antioxidant called quercetin in them). Apples also have Vitamins C, A and Flavonoids, Phosphorus, Iron and Calcium as well as Potassium to help promote heart health.

Weight Management Tips:
- Drink 4-5 bottles of cold water today.
- Get 7-8 hours of sleep; take a 20 minute nap today.

JUICE

Photo Credit: Anusorn Pnachol
FREEDITIGALPHOTOS.NET

WEEK 2, DAY 11
(THE APPLE-CUCUMBER JUICER)

Day 4 of Week 2: Cucumbers and Apples

Add 2 whole cucumbers into a juicer, Add 1 whole apple, Juice until complete, Pour into a glass over ice, if desired or bullet to go blender cup or blender mug, Add ½ cup of 100% orange juice (no pulp), Serve immediately

Health Notes:

Apples – Apples help whiten your teeth by producing saliva, assisting with reducing tooth decay, protects against cancers, gallstones, hemorrhoids, constipation and high cholesterol. They also help you control your weight, prevent cataracts, decrease your chances of developing diabetes and boost your immune system (red apples; which have an antioxidant called quercetin in them). Apples also have Vitamins C, A and Flavonoids, Phosphorus, Iron and Calcium as well as Potassium to help promote heart health.

Cucumbers – Cucumbers are in the family of melons, squash and pumpkins. They are a great source of Vitamins K, C, A and B and are made up 95% water and are great for the eyes, skin and hair due to their anti-inflammatory properties and hair growth stimulation. They also aid in weight loss, digestion and blood pressure control. Cucumbers also dissolve kidney stones and rid the body of waste products.

Weight Management Tips:
- Drink 4-5 bottles of cold water today.
- Get 7-8 hours of sleep; take a 20 minute nap today.
- Have your Juice as breakfast and after your evening workout for best results.
- Do 100 crunches before going to bed (2 sets, 50 each); to burn calories, flatten or to keep your stomach flattened, to build muscle and burn additional calories as you sleep.

SLUSH

Photo Credit: zirconicusso
FREEDIGITALPHOTOS.NET

WEEK 2, DAY 12
(PEACH GRAPE WATERMELON SLUSH)
Day 5 of Week 2: Peaches, Grapes and Watermelon

Add 3 cups of white grapes (or green) into a blender, Add 2 whole watermelon stalks (seed-less), Add ½ cup of frozen peaches (from a bag), Add 1 cup of CRUSHED ice, Blend until thick and smooth, Add ½ cup of chilled 100% apple juice, Pour into a glass or bullet to go blender cup or blender mug, Serve immediately

Health Notes:

Grapes – Grapes originated from Spain and are berries that are similar to blueberries the most. They are power-packed with Vitamins K, C and ripe antioxidants for boosting your health. Grapes also come in various colors; green (white grapes are green grapes), black, pink, yellow, purple and even red. Grapes also heal brain damage, are good for your heart (so that blood can flow through blood vessels more easily) and reduce the cells' ability to store fat, which make them great for weight loss and weight management. They also help fight diabetes, inflammation, skin diseases and aid in muscle health.

Peaches- Peaches are a great fruit that also help fight obesity by keeping you fuller longer; *controlling* your weight. They contribute to keeping your eyes healthy, prevent cancer and hair loss, aid in cleansing your kidneys, bladder and toxins from the body. Also, they are rich in Vitamins A and C as well as a mineral that aids in cell damage protection.

Weight Management Tips:
- Drink 4-5 bottles of cold water today.
- Get 7-8 hours of sleep; take a 20 minute nap today.

JUICE

Photo Credit: Anusorn Pnachol
FREEDIGITALPHOTOS.NET

WEEK 2, DAY 13
(THE CELERY-CUCUMBER JUICER)

Day 6 of Week 2: Celery and Cucumbers

Add 3 celery stalks into a juicer, Add 1 whole cucumber, Juice until complete, Pour into a glass over ice, if desired or bullet to go blender cup or blender mug, Add ½ cup of chilled 100% apple juice, Serve immediately

Health Notes:

Celery- Celery is good for your bone health and fights certain cancers. They also help lower blood pressure, increase blood flow (muscle tissues relaxed throughout the arteries) throughout the body. Celery also helps reduce inflammation, is extremely low in calories, helps improve eye health and digestion.

Cucumbers – Cucumbers are in the family of melons, squash and pumpkins. They are a great source of Vitamins K, C, A and B and are made up 95% water and are great for the eyes, skin and hair due to their anti-inflammatory properties and hair growth stimulation. They also help fight cancers (ovarian, uterine, breast as well as prostate) and aid in weight loss, digestion, blood pressure control, cholesterol reduction and joint pain relief (that is associated with arthritis). Cucumbers also dissolve kidney stones and rid the body of waste products.

Weight Management Tips:
- Drink 4-5 bottles of cold water today.
- Get 7-8 hours of sleep; take a 20 minute nap today.
- Have your Juice as breakfast and after your evening workout for best results.
- Do 100 crunches before going to bed (2 sets, 50 each); to burn calories, flatten or to keep your stomach flattened, to build muscle and burn additional calories as you sleep.

SLUSH

Photo Credit: zirconicusso
FREEDIGITALPHOTOS.NET

WEEK 2, DAY 14
(PINEAPPLE RED-GRAPE SLUSH)
Day 7 of Week 2: Peaches, Pineapples and Red-Grapes

Add 3 cups of red grapes (or green) into a blender, Add 2 whole pineapple stalks, Add 1 cup of peaches, Add 1 cup of CRUSHED ice, Blend until thick and smooth, Add ½ cup of chilled 100% apple juice, Pour into a glass or bullet to go blender cup or blender mug, Serve immediately

Health Notes:

Grapes – Grapes originated from Spain and are berries that are similar to blueberries the most. They are power-packed with Vitamins K, C and ripe antioxidants for boosting your health. Grapes also come in various colors; green (white grapes are green grapes), black, pink, yellow, purple and even red. Grapes also heal brain damage, are good for your heart (so that blood can flow through blood vessels more easily) and reduce the cells' ability to store fat, which make them great for weight loss and weight management.

Peaches- Peaches are a great fruit that also help fight obesity by keeping you fuller longer; *controlling* your weight. They contribute to keeping your eyes healthy, prevent cancer and hair loss, aid in cleansing your kidneys, bladder and toxins from the body. Also, they are rich in Vitamins A and C as well as a mineral that aids in cell damage protection.

Pineapples – Today, the largest producers of pineapples are in Brazil, Costa Rica, the United States, Hawaii and the Philippines. Pineapples are a natural weight loss food and are rich in Vitamin C, Thiamin, copper and boosts the immune system to fight against colds, flu symptoms and other diseases. They also help ease arthritis pain.

Weight Management Tips:
- Drink 4-5 bottles of cold water today.
- Get 7-8 hours of sleep; take a 20 minute nap today.

THE 21 DAY JUICE FAST | HEALTHILY DRINK YOUR WAY THIN

WEEK 3
BEATS WEEK

Photo Credit: Anusorn Pnachol
FREEDIGITALPHOTOS.NET

WEEK 3, DAY 15
(THE ORANGE-BEAT JUICER)

Day 1 of Week 3: Oranges and Beats

Add 2 whole (peeled) oranges into a juicer, Add 1 whole beat, Juice until complete, Pour into a glass over ice, if desired or bullet to go blender cup or blender mug, Add ½ cup of chilled 100% apple juice, Serve immediately

Health Notes:

Oranges- Oranges are rich in potassium and Vitamin C. Oranges help regulate blood pressure, aid in relieving constipation, infections, risk of liver cancer, kidney stones and lowers cholesterol. This fruit is also rich in citrus limonoids, which have proved to fight a number of varieties of cancers inclusive of: skin, lung, breast, stomach and colon.

Beats – Beats cleanse the body and are a tonic for the liver and purifies the blood as well as prevents many forms of cancer. Beats also help reduce depression, high blood pressure, give energy and are a great source of Fiber, Vitamins A, B & C, beta-carotene, Iron, folic acid *(especially for women that are pregnant along with the Vitamin B and Iron)* as well as Potassium and Magnesium. Beats also help you detoxify your body and boost your stamina and bone strength and help fight Alzheimer's disease and inflammation.

Weight Management Tips:
- Drink 4-5 bottles of cold water today.
- Get 7-8 hours of sleep; take a 20 minute nap today.
- Have your Juice as breakfast and after your evening workout for best results.
- Do 100 crunches before going to bed (2 sets, 50 each); to burn calories, flatten or to keep your stomach flattened, to build muscle and burn additional calories as you sleep.

SLUSH

Photo Credit: zirconicusso
FREEDIGITALPHOTOS.NET

WEEK 3, DAY 16
(WATERMELON ACAI-BERRY SLUSH)

Day 2 of Week 3: Watermelon and Acai-Berry Juice

Add 5 whole watermelon stalks into a blender, Add 1 cup of CRUSHED ice, Blend until thick and smooth, Add ½ cup of chilled 100% acai-berry juice, Pour into a glass or bullet to go blender cup or blender mug, Serve immediately

Health Notes:

Watermelon - Watermelon is a plant that is originally from Southern Africa. Its fruit is a special berry that has a ripe source of Vitamins C, A, D, B-12, beta carotene, thiamin and B-6. Iron, Calcium, potassium and magnesium are also included. Watermelon is low in calories and aids in wound healing, stress relief and **quenching cravings** to assist with weight loss.

Acai-Berry- The secret ingredient in this slushie is "Acai Berry" juice. Acai berries are known for aiding in lowering cholesterol levels, increasing overall heart health. The acai **oil** in the berry helps with generating healthy skin and the ***pulp*** in the berry aids in weight loss and fighting obesity. Acai berries also boost energy and mental function.

Weight Management Tips:
- Drink 4-5 bottles of cold water today.
- Get 7-8 hours of sleep; take a 20 minute nap today.

THE 21 DAY JUICE FAST | HEALTHILY DRINK YOUR WAY THIN

JUICE

Photo Credit: Anusorn Pnachol
FREEDITIALPHOTOS.NET

WEEK 3, DAY 17
(THE CUCUMBER-BEAT JUICER)

Day 3 of Week 3: Cucumbers and Beats

Add 1 whole cucumbers into a juicer, Add ½ teaspoon of ginkgo biloba, Add 1 whole beat, Juice until complete, Pour into a glass over ice, if desired or bullet to go blender cup or blender mug, Add ½ cup of chilled 100% apple juice, Serve immediately

Health Notes:

Cucumbers – Cucumbers are in the family of melons, squash and pumpkins. They are a great source of Vitamins K, C, A and B and are made up 95% water and are great for the eyes, skin and hair due to their anti-inflammatory properties and hair growth stimulation. They also help fight cancers (ovarian, uterine, breast as well as prostate) and aid in weight loss, digestion, blood pressure control, cholesterol reduction and joint pain relief (that is associated with arthritis). Cucumbers also dissolve kidney stones and rid the body of waste products.

Beats – Beats cleanse the body and are a tonic for the liver and purifies the blood as well as prevents many forms of cancer. Beats also help reduce depression, high blood pressure, give energy and are a great source of Fiber.

Weight Management Tips:
- Drink 4-5 bottles of cold water today.
- Get 7-8 hours of sleep; take a 20 minute nap today.
- Have your Juice as breakfast and after your evening workout for best results.
- Do 100 crunches before going to bed (2 sets, 50 each); to burn calories, flatten or to keep your stomach flattened, to build muscle and burn additional calories as you sleep.

THE 21 DAY JUICE FAST | HEALTHILY DRINK YOUR WAY THIN

SLUSH

Photo Credit: zirconicusso
FREEDIGITALPHOTOS.NET

WEEK 3, DAY 18
("GO-GREEN" APPLE SLUSH)

Day 4 of Week 3: Green Apples and Apple Juice

Add 3 whole (sliced) green apples into a blender, Add 1 cup of CRUSHED ice, Blend until thick and smooth, Add ½ cup of chilled 100% apple juice, Pour into a glass or bullet to go blender cup or blender mug, Serve immediately

Health Notes:

Apples – Apples help whiten your teeth by producing saliva, assisting with reducing tooth decay, protects against cancers, gallstones, hemorrhoids, constipation and high cholesterol.

Apples also help you control your weight, prevent cataracts, decrease your chances of developing diabetes and boost your immune system (red apples; which have an antioxidant called quercetin in them).

Furthermore, apples also have Vitamins C, A and Flavonoids, Phosphorus, Iron and Calcium as well as Potassium to help promote heart health.

Weight Management Tips:
- Drink 4-5 bottles of cold water today.
- Get 7-8 hours of sleep; take a 20 minute nap today.

THE 21 DAY JUICE FAST | HEALTHILY DRINK YOUR WAY THIN

JUICE

Photo Credit: Anusorn Pnachol
FREEDIGITALPHOTOS.NET

WEEK 3, DAY 19
(THE PEAR-BEAT JUICER)
Day 5 of Week 3: Pears and Beats

Add 2 whole pears into a juicer, Add 1 whole beat, Juice until complete, Pour into a glass over ice, if desired or bullet to go blender cup or blender mug, Add ½ cup of chilled 100% apple juice, Serve immediately

Health Notes:

Pears – Pears are filled with Vitamin C and Iron. They are a great source of fiber, help reduce bad cholesterol in the body, fights cancer, acne and aging and increases energy levels and digestion. Pears also helps restore shine to your hair and prevents frizz.

Beats – Beats cleanse the body and are a tonic for the liver and purifies the blood as well as prevents many forms of cancer. Beats also help reduce depression, high blood pressure, give energy and are a great source of Fiber, Vitamins A, B & C, beta-carotene, Iron, folic acid *(especially for women that are pregnant along with the Vitamin B and Iron)* as well as Potassium and Magnesium. Beats also help you detoxify your body and boost your stamina and bone strength and help fight Alzheimer's disease and inflammation.

Weight Management Tips:
- Drink 4-5 bottles of cold water today.
- Get 7-8 hours of sleep; take a 20 minute nap today.
- Have your Juice as breakfast and after your evening workout for best results.
- Do 100 crunches before going to bed (2 sets, 50 each); to burn calories, flatten or to keep your stomach flattened, to build muscle and burn additional calories as you sleep.

SLUSH

Photo Credit: zirconicusso
FREEDIGITALPHOTOS.NET

WEEK 3, DAY 20
(LEMON-LIME PEAR SLUSH)

Day 6 of Week 3: Lemons, Limes and Pears

Add 2 whole (sliced) pears, Add the zests of a lemon and a lime, Add 2 whole (peeled) lemons into a blender, Add 2 whole (peeled) limes, Add 1 cup of CRUSHED ice, Blend until thick and smooth, Add ½ cup of chilled 100% apple juice, Pour into a glass or bullet to go blender cup or blender mug, Serve immediately

Health Notes:

Limes – Limes are rich in Vitamin C and folate. Interestingly, you may think, the juice, fruit and peel of a lime are used to make medicines and help cure severe diarrhea. Limes also kill germs in the skin, aiding in skin care *(preventing aging);* they ease constipation and help prevent fever, urinary tract and bladder infections, ulcers, heart disease *(lowering bad cholesterol)* and even arthritis.

Lemons – Lemons are a great source of citric acid, Vitamins C, Calcium and even Potassium. They also help fight hair loss, lumps on the skin and hands, high blood pressure, arthritis, constipation, burns, vision loss, excess gas, gallstones, internal bleeding, fevers and indigestion as well as aids in cleansing the teeth and dandruff from the hair. Lemons also helps revitalize your skin and aid in weight loss when mixed with recipes that have water (or ice) and honey in them.

Weight Management Tips:
- Drink 4-5 bottles of cold water today.
- Get 7-8 hours of sleep; take a 20 minute nap today.

JUICE

Photo Credit: Anusorn Pnachol
FREEDIGITALPHOTOS.NET

WEEK 3, DAY 21
(THE LEMON-BEAT JUICER)

Day 7 of Week 3: Lemons and Beats

Add 2 whole beats into a juicer, Add 2 whole (peeled) lemons, Add 1 whole apple *(any color; red, yellow or green)*, Juice until complete, Pour into a glass over ice, if desired or bullet to go blender cup or blender mug, Add ½ cup of chilled 100% apple juice (no pulp), Serve immediately

Health Notes:

Beats – Beats cleanse the body and are a tonic for the liver and purifies the blood as well as prevents many forms of cancer. Beats also help reduce depression, high blood pressure, give energy and are a great source of Fiber, Vitamins A, B & C, beta-carotene, Iron and folic acid.

Lemons – Lemons are a great source of citric acid, Vitamins C, Calcium and even Potassium. They also help fight hair loss, lumps on the skin and hands, high blood pressure, arthritis, constipation, burns, vision loss, excess gas, gallstones, internal bleeding, fevers and indigestion as well as aids in cleansing the teeth and dandruff from the hair. Lemons also helps revitalize your skin and aid in weight loss when mixed with recipes that have water (or ice) and honey in them.

Weight Management Tips:
- Drink 4-5 bottles of cold water today.
- Get 7-8 hours of sleep; take a 20 minute nap today.
- Have your Juice as breakfast and after your evening workout for best results.
- Do 100 crunches before going to bed (2 sets, 50 each); to burn calories, flatten or to keep your stomach flattened, to build muscle and burn additional calories as you sleep.

CONGRATULATIONS ON YOUR NEW YOU!

*Keep up the great work by continuing
on with my two newest books, "The 21 Day Smoothie Fast"
and the "21 Day Salad Fast"*

INDEX OF RECIPES

DAY 1	42		DAY 12	64
DAY 2	44		DAY 13	66
DAY 3	46		DAY 14	68
DAY 4	48		DAY 15	70
DAY 5	50		DAY 16	72
DAY 6	52		DAY 17	74
DAY 7	54		DAY 18	76
DAY 8	56		DAY 19	78
DAY 9	58		DAY 20	80
DAY 10	60		DAY 21	82
DAY 11	62			

www.ingramcontent.com/pod-product-compliance
Lightning Source LLC
Chambersburg PA
CBHW071842090426
42811CB00035B/2304/J